Juicing For Liver Health

A Guide to Natural Detox and Wellness

By

Vanessa S. Castaneda

Table of Contents

Introduction

In the quest for robust health and vitality, the liver serves as the body's primary cleansing organ. Maintaining good liver health is essential for overall well-being considering its complex collection of functions, which range from toxin filtering to nutrient metabolization. Juicing, with its wealth of nutrient-dense fruits, vegetables, and herbs, has emerged as a promising natural method for maintaining liver health.

However, harnessing the potential of juicing for liver health entails more than simply mixing components. It comprises a thoughtful and planned approach that takes into account the liver's individual needs and how best to support its functioning through a targeted diet. Monitoring your health and changing your juicing methods might help you realize the full potential of fresh juices to nourish and revitalize your liver.

In this tutorial, we'll look at the science of juicing for liver health, exploring the key nutrients, ingredients, and strategies that can help with detoxification, inflammation reduction, and support overall liver function. From selecting the right components to incorporating juicing into your daily routine, we'll provide practical insights and recommendations to help you start your journey to liver fitness.

Chapter 1: Understanding Liver Health

Introduction to Liver Functions and the Value of Liver Health

The liver, an important component of our digestive system, is required for life support and overall wellness. It is the body's largest solid organ, situated under the rib cage on the right side of the abdomen. The liver performs about 500 essential tasks that aid in the body's metabolic, detoxifying, and regulatory processes. Understanding these functions and the importance of maintaining liver health is fundamental to our well-being.

The Liver Essential Roles

1. **Detoxification**: The liver filters and eliminates toxins from the blood, such as metabolic wastes, medications, alcohol, and environmental pollutants.

2. **Metabolism**: It plays a crucial role in metabolizing carbs, proteins, and fats, transforming them into energy and essential components for the organism. The liver contributes to stable glucose levels by turning excess glucose into glycogen for storage and releasing it back into the bloodstream as needed.

3. **Protein Synthesis**: The liver produces a variety of proteins, including albumin (which regulates blood volume and pressure) and the clotting factors required for blood coagulation.

4. **Production and Excretion of Bile**: The liver produces bile, which aids in the absorption and digestion of fats and fat-soluble vitamins (A, D, E, and K) in the intestine

5. **Vitamin and Mineral Storage**: It stores vitamins A, D, E, K, and B12, along with minerals such as iron and copper, and releases them as the body needs them.

6. **Cholesterol Management**: The liver produces cholesterol and proteins that aid in the transport of fats through the body. It also plays a crucial role in turning excess cholesterol into bile acids, which are eventually removed from the body.

7. **Immune System Support**: The liver is part of the immune system; it contains Kupffer cells that digest bacteria, fungi, and other pathogens.

Importance of Liver Health

Given the liver's vital functions, its health is important to our body's ability to function properly. Liver diseases such as hepatitis, fatty liver disease, cirrhosis, and liver cancer can substantially affect these functions, resulting in serious health consequences or even death. Excessive alcohol intake, obesity, infections, and exposure to toxic substances are all risk factors for liver disease.

A balanced diet high in fruits, vegetables, and whole grains, moderate exercise, a reduction in alcohol intake, and abstaining from liver-damaging chemicals are all necessary to maintain liver health. Frequent checkups can help detect liver issues early, increasing the likelihood that treatment will be successful.

In summary- The liver's numerous functions in detoxification, metabolism, and control are indispensable for maintaining health. Recognizing the significance of liver health and adopting proactive measures to maintain this crucial organ can result in a healthier, more vibrant life. By supporting our liver, we help our body cleanse itself, digest food, manage energy, and much more, emphasizing the liver's role as a cornerstone of our overall well-being and health.

Typical Liver Disease

Liver diseases and ailments affect the liver's capacity to carry out essential tasks, potentially leading to major health issues. Here are some of the most frequent liver disorders and conditions:

Fatty Liver Disease

Fatty liver disease is defined by the accumulation of fat in liver cells. It primarily falls into two categories:

- Non-alcoholic fatty liver disease (NAFLD) is frequently related to obesity, diabetes, and metabolic syndrome. NAFLD can progress to non-alcoholic steatohepatitis (NASH), a more serious condition that can result in cirrhosis or liver cancer.
- Alcoholic Liver Disease (ALD): Excessive alcohol use causes fat buildup, inflammation, and, finally, cirrhosis.

Hepatitis

Hepatitis is an inflammation of the liver caused by viral infections, poisons (such as alcohol and some drugs), and autoimmune illnesses. The most prevalent kinds of viral hepatitis include the following:

- Hepatitis A: Frequently transmitted through the use of contaminated food or water.
- Hepatitis B: Spreads by contact with contaminated bodily fluids like blood, sperm, or vaginal secretions.
- Hepatitis C: Hepatitis C is primarily transmitted via blood-to-blood contact, such as sharing needles or from mother to child during childbirth.

Cirrhosis

Cirrhosis is the advanced stage of scarring (fibrosis) of the liver caused by a variety of liver diseases and disorders, including hepatitis and chronic drinking. Each time the liver is wounded, it attempts to mend itself, resulting in scar tissue. As the disease advances, the liver's capacity to function deteriorates.

Liver Cancer

Primary liver cancer starts in the liver. The prevalent variety is hepatocellular carcinoma

(HCC), which frequently manifests in individuals with long-term liver conditions such as cirrhosis caused by infection with hepatitis B or C.

Autoimmune Liver Disease

These disorders arise when the body's immune system attacks the liver, producing inflammation and damage. Here are several examples:

- Autoimmune Hepatitis: A chronic illness that can progress to cirrhosis and liver failure if not addressed.
- Primary Biliary Cholangitis (PBC) and Primary Sclerosing Cholangitis (PSC) are diseases affecting the liver's bile ducts, resulting in severe liver damage and cirrhosis.

Gilbert's Syndrome

A minor liver condition in which the liver does not adequately handle bilirubin. It's normally harmless and doesn't need to be treated.

Hemochromatosis

Iron accumulates in the body, including the liver. Excess iron can cause liver damage, cirrhosis, and even liver cancer over time.

The liver's health is significant to overall wellness. Many liver diseases can be prevented or managed with early detection and proper care, which may include lifestyle modifications, medications, or, in extreme cases, surgery. Regular health check-ups, maintaining a healthy lifestyle, and avoiding risk factors can help preserve liver health and disease prevention.

Lifestyle Factors Affecting Liver Health

Lifestyle factors play a substantial role in influencing liver health. Positive habits can help the liver function, while negative ones can lead to liver damage over time. Understanding and modifying these factors can help prevent liver disease and maintain overall well-being. Here are some of the key lifestyle factors that influence liver health:

Alcohol Consumption: Excess alcohol use is the major cause of liver damage. Alcohol can damage liver cells, and lead to conditions such as fatty liver, alcoholic hepatitis, fibrosis, and cirrhosis. Alcohol use should be limited or abstain entirely for the sake of liver health.

Diet and Nutrition: Poor dietary choices can contribute to liver difficulties.

- High-fat, sugary, and processed foods can cause fat to accumulate in the liver, a condition known as non-alcoholic fatty liver disease (NAFLD).
- A balanced diet rich in fruits, vegetables, lean protein, and whole grains promotes liver health by supplying essential nutrients and antioxidants that help neutralize toxins.

Obesity and Physical Inactivity: Obesity, particularly excessive belly fat, is closely linked to NAFLD and its more severe form, non-alcoholic steatohepatitis (NASH). Engaging in Regular physical activity and maintaining a healthy weight through diet and exercise are essential to preventing fat accumulation in the liver and supporting overall liver function.

Smoking: Not only does smoking increase the risk of liver cancer, but it also exacerbates the negative consequences of other risk factors for liver disease, such as alcohol intake and obesity. Quitting smoking benefits both liver health and overall well-being.

Drug and Medication Overuse: Both illegal drug use and the abuse of prescription and over-the-counter medications can harm the liver. For example, chronic acetaminophen (Tylenol) use is a common cause of abrupt liver failure. It is important to use medications exactly as prescribed and avoid using illegal drugs.

Toxic Exposure: Regular exposure to environmental toxins and chemicals, such as those found in cleaning products, pesticides, and industrial chemicals, can cause liver damage in the long run. Wearing protective gear and limiting exposure to harmful substances can help protect liver health.

Stress: Chronic stress can indirectly affect liver health by encouraging harmful behaviors such as overeating, excessive alcohol consumption, and ignoring physical activity. Handling stress through procedures such as exercise, meditation, or counseling can support general health, including liver function.

In summary- Liver health is significantly influenced by lifestyle choices. Embracing a healthy lifestyle that includes a balanced diet, frequent physical activity, reasonable alcohol consumption, not smoking, managing medication and toxin exposure, infection prevention, and stress reduction can help preserve liver function and prevent liver disease. Making these positive changes not only endorses the liver but also enhances overall health and quality of life.

Chapter 2: Diet's Impact on Liver Health

Overview of How Diet Impacts Liver Health

Diet plays an important part in liver health, influencing its function and risk of illness. The liver is integral to different metabolic processes, including the metabolism of fats, proteins, and carbohydrates, as well as the detoxification of toxic substances. A balanced diet assists the liver in performing these functions effectively, while a bad diet can lead to liver damage over time. Here is an outline of how diet influences liver health:

Positive Dietary Impacts on Liver Health

1. A diet rich in fruits, vegetables, whole grains, lean protein, and healthy fats can subsidize liver function and lower the risk of liver disease. These meals provide essential nutrients, antioxidants, and fiber, which help retain optimal liver health.

2. Fruits and vegetables are high in antioxidants and phytonutrients, which help reduce inflammation and protect liver cells from harm. Leafy greens, berries, and cruciferous vegetables (such as broccoli and Brussels sprouts) are especially healthy.

3. Whole grains, such as oats, barley, and quinoa, provide dietary fiber, which helps to control blood sugar levels and lessen the risk of fatty liver disease.

4. Lean protein sources such as fish, poultry, beans, and lentils assist liver function without adding excessive fat to the diet.

5. Healthy fats, especially those rich in omega-3 fatty acids found in fish, nuts, and seeds, can help lower liver fat, inflammation, and the risk of nonalcoholic fatty liver disease (NAFLD).

Negative Dietary Influences on Liver Health

6. High intake of saturated and trans fats, typically found in processed foods, fast food, and fatty cuts of meat, can lead to

fat accumulation in the liver, contributing to NAFLD and its progression.

7. Excessive consumption of refined carbs and sugars, such as those found in sugary drinks, sweets, and white bread, can increase liver fat, leading to NAFLD.

8. Alcohol is metabolized by the liver and can result in damage to liver cells, leading to fatty liver, alcoholic hepatitis, fibrosis, and cirrhosis with excessive consumption.

9. High salt consumption can contribute to liver damage and worsen the condition of those already suffering from liver disease by encouraging water retention and swelling.

Dietary Recommendations for Liver Health

I.   Adopt a Mediterranean-style diet that emphasizes fruits, vegetables, whole grains, legumes, nuts, lean proteins, and healthy fats.

II. Limit your intake of added sugars and refined carbohydrates: Avoid sugary drinks and snacks; choose whole fruits and complex carbohydrates.

III. Reduce saturated and trans fats by choosing lean cuts of meat and low-fat dairy products, as well as avoiding fried and processed foods.

IV. Moderate alcohol consumption: Those who consume alcohol should do so in moderation or abstain completely, especially if they have a history of liver illness.

V. Stay hydrated: Drinking enough water is essential for helping the liver process and remove waste products.

A well-balanced diet not only supports liver health but also contributes to overall well-being. Individuals can significantly influence their liver's health and function by adopting thoughtful dietary choices.

Essential Nutrient for Liver Health.

The liver is a complex organ that plays an important role in metabolizing nutrients, detoxifying toxic substances, and conducting hundreds of other essential functions. Certain nutrients are particularly important for endorsing liver health and optimizing its functions. Incorporating foods rich in these nutrients can help maintain liver health and prevent liver damage. Here are the key nutrients essential for liver function:

1. Omega-3 Fatty Acids

Omega-3 fatty acids, found in fish like salmon, sardines, and mackerel, as well as flaxseeds, chia seeds, and walnuts, are essential for liver health. They help reduce inflammation and are linked to a lower risk of nonalcoholic fatty liver disease (NAFLD).

2. Fiber

Dietary fiber, particularly in fruits, vegetables, whole grains, and legumes, helps restrain blood sugar levels and can lower the risk of fatty liver disease. Fiber aids in digestion and helps maintain a healthy weight, which is essential for liver health.

3. Vitamins

Vitamin D: There is growing evidence that vitamin D plays a role in liver health, with deficits associated with a variety of liver illnesses, including NAFLD. Vitamin D can be gained through sun exposure, fatty fish, and fortified meals.

Vitamin E: Known for its antioxidant properties, vitamin E can aid in protecting the liver from harm. Those with NAFLD really benefit from it. Nuts, seeds, spinach, and broccoli are good sources.

Vitamin C: Another powerful antioxidant, vitamin C helps protect liver cells from oxidative stress. Citrus fruits, berries, kiwi, bell peppers, and tomatoes are also good sources.

B vitamins are essential for metabolizing alcohol and other toxins, and they play an important role in liver function. Whole grains, nuts, seeds, dairy products, and leafy green vegetables are all sources of these nutrients.

4. Antioxidants

Antioxidants such as glutathione, selenium, and zinc protect the liver by neutralizing harmful free radicals. Glutathione is produced by the liver and can be boosted by consuming sulfur-rich foods such as garlic, onions, and cruciferous vegetables. Selenium and zinc can be found in nuts, seeds, shellfish, and meat.

5. Amino Acids

Amino acids, the protein building blocks, are necessary for detoxification processes and repairing liver tissue. Amino acids can be found in meat, fish, tofu, lentils, and dairy products.

Certain amino acids, such as methionine and cysteine, aid with the production of glutathione.

6. Choline

Choline is crucial for liver function, as it helps transport fat from the liver to cells throughout the body. A choline shortage can cause fat accumulation in the liver. Eggs, liver, peanuts, and soybeans are rich in choline.

Incorporating a Balanced Diet: A diet high in these nutrients can benefit liver health, lower the risk of liver disease, and improve the liver's detoxification capacity. It is important to consume a variety of nutrient-dense foods to cover the wide range of nutrients required for liver function. In some circumstances, particularly if there is a danger of deficiency, dietary supplements may be recommended; however, it is best to check with a healthcare physician before beginning any supplement regimen.

Foods to Avoid for Optimal Liver Health

For optimal liver health, you must be attentive to your diet, since certain foods and chemicals can stress or harm the liver over time. Here are certain meals and beverages you should limit or avoid.

1. **Alcohol**: Excessive alcohol consumption is a major cause of liver injury. It can cause fatty liver disease, alcoholic hepatitis, fibrosis, and cirrhosis.

2. **Added Sugars**: High consumption of added sugars, such as high-fructose corn syrup found in soft drinks, sweets, and baked goods, can cause fat accumulation in the liver, resulting in nonalcoholic fatty liver disease (NAFLD).

3. **Refined Carbohydrates**: White bread, white rice, and pasta prepared with refined flour can have a similar impact to added sweets, spiking blood sugar and insulin

levels and contributing to liver fat accumulation.

4. **Fried and Fast Food**: Fried fast foods are high in calories and trans fats, and they lead to weight gain and obesity, both of which are substantial risk factors for NAFLD.

5. **Red and Processed Meats**: High in saturated fat, these can increase the risk of NAFLD and worsen liver health. It has been suggested to limit consumption of foods such as bacon, sausages, and fatty cuts of beef or pork.

6. **Salt:** Excessive salt intake can lead to water retention and worsen illnesses such as cirrhosis, where the liver's capacity to function is significantly damaged. Processed foods are a main source of dietary sodium.

7. **Supplements and Herbal Remedies:** High amounts of vitamin A, for example,

can harm the liver. Some herbal supplements, including kava, comfrey, and Chinese herbs, have been related to liver disease.

8. **Sugary Snacks and Beverages:** Sweets, cakes, and sugary drinks can all contribute to liver fat accumulation. Whole fruits and other natural sources of sugar are better for liver health

General Recommendations:

It's important to stay hydrated when drinking lots of water, which facilitates the liver's easier toxin removal.

Focus on Whole Foods: A diet high in fruits, vegetables, whole grains, and lean proteins can help liver health and lower the risk of liver disease.

Do Regular Exercise: Physical activity promotes the use of triglycerides as fuel and can help reduce liver fat.

A balanced diet rich in nutrients and low in processed foods, combined with regular physical activity, not only promotes liver health but also helps general well-being. If you have liver disease or are at risk of acquiring it, speak with a healthcare provider or a dietitian for personalized guidance.

Chapter 3: The Basics of Juicing

Introduction to Juicing: Unlocking the Nutritional Potential of Fresh Produce

Juicing has emerged as a popular trend in the realm of nutrition and wellness, offering a convenient and flavorful way to improve our intake of fruits and vegetables. It involves extracting the liquid content and nutrients from fresh produce, leaving behind the pulp, resulting in a concentrated and readily digestible beverage. In this introduction to juicing, we'll explore its advantages, practical tips for getting started, and how it can improve your general health and well-being.

Advantages of Juicing

1. **Nutrient Density:** Juicing allows you to consume a large quantity of fruits and vegetables in concentrated form, providing a rich source of vitamins, minerals, and antioxidants that are required for good health.

2. **Easy Digestion**: Eliminating the fiber during the juicing process facilitates the body's absorption of nutrients, providing a rapid and effective means of nourishing your cells.

3. **Hydration**: Juices are an excellent way to stay hydrated, particularly for those who find it difficult to consume enough water throughout the day.

4. **Variety and Flavour**: Juicing opens up a new world of flavor combinations, allowing you to experiment with various fruits, vegetables, and herbs to make tasty and refreshing beverages.

5. **Detoxification**: Some proponents claim that juicing can help the body's natural detoxification processes by providing a concentrated amount of nutrients that improve liver function and boost toxin removal.

Advice for Beginning Juicing Journey:

a. **Choose Quality Produce**: Choose fresh, organic fruits and vegetables whenever feasible to maximize the nutritional value of your juice. Wash properly before juicing to remove any dirt or pesticide residues.

b. **Invest in a Good Juicer**: Consider purchasing a high-quality juicer that suits your demands and fits your budget. Centrifugal juicers are best for beginners, due to their inexpensive and simple use, while masticating juicers offer higher juice results and maintain more nutrients.

c. **Balance Your Ingredients**: Aim for a balanced ratio of fruits and vegetables in your juice to avoid unreasonable sugar consumption. Include a variety of colors and varieties of produce to guarantee a various collection of nutrients.

d. **Start Simple**: Begin with simple juice recipes that include recognizable ingredients such as carrots, apples, spinach, and cucumbers before trying more exotic flavors and combinations.

e. **Drink Right Away**: Freshly squeezed juice should be consumed immediately to maintain its nutritional value and flavor. If preserving juice for later use, keep it refrigerated in an airtight container and eat it within 24 hours.

f. **Mindful Consumption**: Juicing can be a nutritious supplement to your diet, but it should not be used to replace full fruits and vegetables or other vital food groups. It can be used to supplement a well-balanced and varied diet.

Juicing is a tasty and easy way to increase your consumption of essential nutrients and improve your general health and well-being. Incorporating colorful, fresh vegetables into your daily diet will help you nourish your body from the inside out, encouraging longevity and vigor. Juicing can be a joyful and fulfilling aspect of your healthy lifestyle if you have the proper tools, materials, and mindset. So gather your favorite fruits and veggies, turn on the juicer, and start making juice!

Choosing the Right Juicer

Choosing the perfect juicer is determined by your interests, lifestyle, and budget. There are various types of juicers on the market, each with its own distinct features and benefits. Here's an overview of the different types of juicers and the elements to consider while making your choice:

1. Centrifugal Juicer

How it Works: To extract juice from fruits and vegetables, these juicers use centrifugal force. They have a fast-spinning blade that shreds produce, separating the juice and pulp.

Pros: Quick juice extraction process.
more cheap than other types of juicers.
simple to clean and build.

Cons: Heat may destroy some nutrients and enzymes.
less effective in obtaining juice from leafy greens and wheatgrass.

Best for: beginners, those with limited time, and those on a budget who choose speed and convenience over maximal nutrient retention.

2. Masticating Juicers (Cold Press or Slow Juicers)

How it works: To extract juice from fruits and vegetables, these juicers crush them slowly. They crush and press produce to extract the juice, which results in better nutritional retention.

Pros: Slowly, juice preserves nutrients and enzymes. consistently extracts juice from fiber produce, including leafy greens and wheatgrass. suitable for making nut milk, sorbets, and baby food.

Cons: The juicer processing is slower than with centrifugal juicers.
typically more expensive.
Cleaning and assembly take longer.

Best for: health aficionados, those looking for maximum nutrient retention, and people who value adaptability and are ready to invest in a higher-quality juicer.

3. Twin Gear Juicers

How it works: These juicers employ two interlocking gears to smash and press fruits and vegetables, producing juice with little heat and oxidation.

Pros: high juice output and nutrient retention. versatile, able to juice a wide range of produce, including leafy greens, hard vegetables, and wheatgrass.
Create an extremely dry pulp, suggesting efficient extraction.

Cons: Expensive investment.
bigger and heavier than other juicers.
more difficult to assemble and clean.

Best for: serious juicers, health-conscious people, and those who value optimal vitamin preservation and juice yield.

Factors to Consider

- **Budget**: Decide how much you're willing to spend on a juicer. Centrifugal juicers are often less expensive than masticating or twin-gear juicers.
- **Type of Produce**: Consider the type of fruits and veggies you'll be juicing the most. If you intend to juice a lot of leafy greens or wheatgrass, a masticating or dual-gear juicer would be more suitable.
- **Cleaning**: Look for juicers with removable parts that can be washed in the dishwasher or by hand. Complicated cleaning procedures can discourage regular juicing.
- **Juice Quality**: Consider the quality of the juices generated by the juicer, such as flavor, texture, and nutrient content.

Choosing the best juicer is a personal decision based on your specific preferences and priorities. When making your decision, consider your budget, ease of cleaning, juice quality, and the type of produce you'll be juicing the most. Whether you choose a centrifugal juicer for speed and convenience or a masticating or twin-gear juicer for optimal nutrient retention, the proper juicer will enable you to enjoy fresh, nutritious juices as part of your healthy lifestyle.

Shopping and Storage Tips for Fresh Produce

Shopping for fresh produce is crucial for juicing because the quality of your ingredients has a direct impact on the flavor and nutritional value of your juice. Here are some shopping and storing suggestions to get the most out of your fruit.

Shopping Tip:

I. **Select Seasonal Produce**: Seasonal fruits and vegetables are typically fresher, tastier, and less expensive. Check what is in season in your area and incorporate it into your juices.

II. **Look for Freshness Signs**: Choose produce that is firm, bright in color, and devoid of bruises, blemishes, or rotting.

Avoid fruits and vegetables with mold, soft areas, or pungent odors.

III. **Buy Organic When Possible**: Choose organic vegetables, particularly those on the Environmental Working Group's "Dirty Dozen" list, which are more likely to have pesticide residues.

IV. **Buy in Bulk to Save Money**: Purchase bigger amounts of fruits and vegetables when they are in season or on sale, then freeze or juice them for later use.

V. **Go to Farmers' Markets or Local Farms**: Support local farmers and artisans by shopping at farmer's markets or participating in a community-supported agriculture (CSA) program. You'll frequently find fresher vegetables and uncommon types that are not accessible in supermarkets.

Storage Tips:

VI. **Refrigerate Properly**: To keep most fruits and vegetables fresh, store them in the refrigerator. Some goods, such as tomatoes, avocados, bananas, and citrus fruits, can be stored at room temperature until mature and then refrigerated.

VII. **Keep Produce Dry**: Moisture causes fruits and vegetables to decay faster. Store produce in perforated plastic bags or breathable containers to promote air circulation and prevent moisture buildup.

VIII. **Separate Ethylene Producers**: Some fruits, such as apples, bananas, and tomatoes, create ethylene gas, which can speed up the ripening and deterioration of other produce. Keep ethylene-producing fruits separate from ethylene-sensitive foods such as leafy greens and berries.

IX. **Properly Store Leafy Greens**: Remove any bands or ties from leafy greens, wash and dry completely, then wrap them in paper towels and place them in a breathable container or plastic bag in the refrigerator's crisper drawer.

X. **Freeze Excess Produce**: If you have leftover fruits and veggies that you won't be able to use before they spoil, freeze them for future use in smoothies or juices. Cut or slice the vegetables into manageable pieces, put them out on a baking sheet to freeze separately, and then move them to freezer bags or containers.

Following these shopping and storage techniques will guarantee that your fresh produce stays fresh and flavorful, allowing you to drink wonderful and nutritious juices every day.

Chapter 4: Juicing Ingredients for Liver Health

Detailed Information on Fruits, Vegetables, and Herbs Beneficial for the Liver

Here's a comprehensive list of fruits, vegetables, and herbs that are good for liver health:

Fruits;

a. **Berries**: Blueberries, strawberries, raspberries, and blackberries are rich in antioxidants like anthocyanins, which help reduce inflammation and protect liver cells from harm.

b. **Citrus Fruits**: Citrus fruits such as oranges, lemons, grapefruits, and limes are rich in vitamin C and flavonoids, which stimulate liver detoxification enzymes and promote liver health.

c. **Apples**: Packed with pectin and antioxidants, apples aid in detoxification and blood sugar regulation, lowering the risk of fatty liver disease.

d. **Kiwi**: Rich in vitamin C, kiwi helps neutralize free radicals and boosts the liver's antioxidant defenses, supporting detoxification and general liver function.

e. **Grapes**: They include resveratrol and other antioxidants that preserve liver cells and may help prevent fatty liver disease.

f. **Pineapple**: Pineapple contains bromelain, an enzyme that helps with digestion and liver cleansing. Pineapples also include antioxidants like vitamin C and manganese.

Vegetables:

g. **Leafy Greens**: Kale, spinach, Swiss chard, and other leafy greens are high in chlorophyll, which helps to cleanse and detoxify the liver. They also include antioxidants and fiber, which aid in liver function.

h. **Cruciferous Vegetables**: Broccoli, Brussels sprouts, cauliflower, and cabbage contain sulfur compounds that aid liver detoxification pathways. They also include antioxidants and fiber, which promote liver function.

i. **Beets**: Beets are rich in betaine and antioxidants, which help protect liver cells from harm and stimulate detoxification. They also stimulate bile synthesis, which aids in fat digestion.

j. **Carrots**: High in beta-carotene and other antioxidants, carrots aid in reducing inflammation and improving liver function. They also include fiber, which helps with digestion and toxin disposal.

k. **Artichokes**: These vegetables have cynarin and silymarin, which help to maintain liver function by boosting the generation of bile and shielding liver cells from harm.

l. **Turmeric**: This spice has curcumin, a powerful antioxidant and anti-inflammatory that helps the liver function by lowering oxidative stress and inflammation.

Herbs:

m. **Milk Thistle**: contains silymarin, a powerful antioxidant and anti-inflammatory substance that protects liver cells and promotes regeneration.

n. **Dandelion Root**: Helps liver detoxification by increasing bile production and aiding toxin removal from the body.

o. **Ginger**: Ginger contains gingerol, a substance with anti-inflammatory and antioxidant effects that promotes liver health and digestion.

p. **Peppermint**: Enhances liver and gallbladder function by increasing bile flow and facilitating digestion.

q. **Licorice Root**: Contains glycyrrhizin, a substance that helps liver function by lowering inflammation and facilitating detoxification.

r. **Burdock Root**: Helps with liver cleansing and blood purification by boosting the elimination of toxins from the body.

Including a range of these fruits, vegetables, and herbs in your diet can aid in detoxification, inflammation reduction, and liver health support. It's crucial to eat them as part of a well-balanced diet full of whole foods and to speak with a doctor before making any big dietary changes, particularly if you already have liver problems.

The Science Behind How These Nutrients Promote Liver Health.

The listed ingredients—fruits, vegetables, and herbs—contain a variety of chemicals that promote liver health via a variety of processes. Here's the science behind how certain substances promote liver health:

Antioxidants

- **Berries, Citrus Fruits, and Grapes**: Contains vitamin C, flavonoids, and anthocyanins, which neutralize free radicals and reduce oxidative stress and inflammation in the liver.

- **Apples, Kiwi**: Packed with antioxidants, including quercetin and vitamin C, which protect liver cells from toxins and oxidative stress.

Fiber:

- **Leafy Greens, Cruciferous Vegetables, Beets: These high-fiber veggies promote regular** bowel movements and aid in the evacuation of toxins from the body, which benefits liver health.
- **Carrots**: High-fiber carrots help manage blood sugar levels, lowering the risk of fatty liver disease and insulin resistance.

Phytonutrients

- **Cruciferous Vegetables**: They have sulfur-containing chemicals, such as glucosinolates, that help liver detoxification pathways and improve the liver's capacity to get rid of toxins.
- **Turmeric**: Contains curcumin, a strong anti-inflammatory substance that helps

lessen hepatic inflammation & protect liver cells from harm.

Bile Production and Flow

- **Artichokes**: Contain compounds like cynarin and silymarin, which boost bile production and flow, aiding in digestion and toxin clearance in the liver.
- **Dandelion Roots**: Promotes bile synthesis and flow, which improves the liver's detoxification abilities.

Anti-inflammatory Substances

- **Turmeric and Ginger**: These foods have strong anti-inflammatory qualities due to the presence of substances like curcumin and gingerol, which lessen liver inflammation and shield liver cells from harm.
- **Milk Thistle**: This herb shields liver cells from oxidative stress and toxicity by containing silymarin, a potent antioxidant and anti-inflammatory substance.

Liver Detoxification

- **Dandelion Root and Burdock Root**: They help eliminate toxins, improve liver function, and promote general health.
- **Licorice Root**: It contains glycyrrhizin, a substance that improves liver function by lowering inflammation and facilitating detoxification.

Overall Nutritional Support

- **All Mentioned Ingredients**: Provide vital vitamins, minerals, and nutrients that promote liver health, such as vitamin C, vitamin E, beta-carotene, and several B vitamins.

By including these substances in your diet, you can improve liver health by reducing inflammation, boosting detoxification, and protecting liver cells from toxins and oxidative stress. To maximize the beneficial benefits of the liver, a balanced diet should include a range of fruits, vegetables, and herbs.

Tips for Preparing Ingredients to Maintain Their Nutritional Worth

To preserve the nutritional content of juicing materials, particularly fruits, vegetables, and herbs, they must be handled appropriately during preparation. Here are some pointers to help you maintain the nutritional content of your ingredients:

Choose Fresh, High-Quality Produce

- Ripe, fresh food has the highest concentrations of antioxidants, vitamins, and minerals. Choose it as soon as possible.
- To minimize your exposure to pesticides and other chemicals, choose organic vegetables.

Wash thoroughly

- Rinse fruits and vegetables with cold water to remove dirt, bacteria, and pesticide residues.

- Use a vegetable brush to thoroughly wash firm produce, such as carrots and potatoes.

Minimal Processing

- Avoid cutting, slicing, and peeling to prevent nutrient loss. Fruit and vegetable skins should be left on if feasible since they often contain vital nutrients and fiber.
- Cut produce right before juicing to reduce exposure to air and maintain freshness.

Proper Storage

- Keep produce in the refrigerator or a cool, dark spot to prevent nutrient breakdown.
- Keep leafy greens fresh and crispy by storing them in perforated plastic bags or ventilated containers.

Juice Immediately

- While preparing vegetables and fruits, juice them right away to prevent vitamin loss. The highest concentrations of vitamins, minerals, and enzymes can be found in freshly squeezed juice.

- If juice needs to be refrigerated for later use, put it into an airtight container and use it within a day.

Use Cold Press or Masticating Juicers

- These types of juicers minimize heat and oxidation, which can lead to the degradation of nutrients and enzymes, by operating at reduced speeds.
- These juicers extract juice more slowly, but they also retain more of the nutrients from the components.

Drink Freshly Juice

- Consume freshly juiced fruits and vegetables as soon as possible for the best vitamin absorption and health benefits.
- Allowing juice to sit for an extended time may cause it to lose nutritional value.

Utilize Juice Pulp

- Use leftover pulp in recipes like soups, smoothies, or baked goods to reduce waste and increase nutritional intake.
- The pulp provides fiber and other nutrients that can boost the nutritional value of your food.

By following these guidelines, you can ensure that your ingredients maintain their optimum nutritional worth, allowing you to reap the full advantages of fresh, nutrient-dense juice. Remember that integrating a variety of fruits, vegetables, and herbs into your diet is essential for maintaining overall health and wellness.

Chapter 5: Liver-Healing Juice Recipes

A Collection of Juicing Recipes for Liver Wellness

Here's a compilation of juicing recipes specifically designed to improve liver health by including fruits, vegetables, and herbs known for their liver-healthy properties:

Liver Cleanse Green Juice

Ingredients:

- 1 cucumber

- 2 celery stalks

- 1 cup of kale

- 1 handful spinach

- 1/2 lemon, peeled

- 1-inch slice of ginger

Directions:

- Thoroughly wash all the ingredients
- Cut the cucumber and celery into smaller pieces if necessary.
- Put all the ingredients in your juicer.
- Process the juice until smooth.
- Before serving, stir it

Nutritional Benefits:

Cucumbers and celery provide hydration and antioxidants that aid in liver cleansing.
Kale and spinach are rich in chlorophyll and antioxidants, which promote liver health and cleansing.
Lemon and ginger provide antioxidants and anti-inflammatory compounds that help the liver function.

Citrus Beet Liver Detox Juice

Ingredients:

- 1 medium peeled beet

- 2 peeled oranges

- 1/2 lemon, peeled

- 1-inch slice of ginger

Directions:

- Thoroughly wash all the ingredients
- Peel the beets, oranges, and lemons.
- Cut the beetroot into smaller pieces if necessary.
- Combine all the ingredients in your juicer.
- Process the juice until smooth.
- Before serving, stir it

Nutritional Benefits:

Beets are a good source of betaine, which helps with bile production and liver detoxification.
Oranges and lemons have significant levels of vitamin C and flavonoids, which protect liver cells and stimulate detoxification.
Ginger contains anti-inflammatory qualities that promote liver health.

Carrot Apple Ginger Liver Tonic

Ingredients:

- 3 carrots

- 2 apples, cored

- 1-inch slice of ginger

Directions:

- Thoroughly wash all the ingredients
- Core the apples
- Peel the ginger
- Combine all the ingredients in your juicer.
- Process juice until smooth.
- Before serving, stir it.

Nutritional Benefits:

Carrots are rich in beta-carotene and antioxidants that support liver health and detoxification.

Apples include pectin, which aids in toxin removal from the digestive tract.

Ginger has anti-inflammatory and digestive properties, which promote overall liver function.

Turmeric Liver Detox Elixir

Ingredients:

- 2 carrots

- 1 peeled Orange

- 1/2 peeled lemon

- 1-inch turmeric root

- 1/4 teaspoon of black pepper (improves curcumin absorption)

Directions:

- Thoroughly wash all the ingredients
- Peel carrots, oranges, lemons, and turmeric root.
- Combine all the ingredients in your juicer.
- Process juice until smooth.
- Before serving, stir it.

Nutritional Benefits:

Carrots and oranges have significant levels of vitamin C and antioxidants, which promote liver health and detoxification.

Turmeric includes curcumin, a potent anti-inflammatory that improves liver function and protects liver cells from harm.

Black pepper boosts curcumin absorption, which improves its efficiency.

Beetroot Liver Cleanse Juice

Ingredients:

- 1 peeled beet

- 1 cored green apple

- 2 carrots

- 1/2 lemon, peeled

- 1-inch slice of ginger

Directions:

- Wash all components thoroughly.

- Peel the beets, lemons, and ginger.
- Cut the beetroot into smaller pieces if necessary.
- Combine all the ingredients in your juicer.
- Process juice until smooth.
- Before serving, stir it.

Nutritional Benefits:

Beets are a good source of betaine, which helps with bile production and liver detoxification.
Lemon and ginger provide antioxidants and anti-inflammatory compounds that help the liver function. Apples include pectin, which aids in toxin removal from the digestive tract. Carrots are rich in beta-carotene and antioxidants that support liver health and detoxification.

Pineapple Cilantro Liver Flush Juice

Ingredients:

- 2 cups chunky pineapple

- 1/2 cucumber

- 1/2 cup of raw cilantro

- 1/2 lemon, peeled

Directions:

- Wash all ingredients thoroughly.
- Cut the pineapple into small slices.
- Peel the cucumbers and lemons.
- Combine all the ingredients in your juicer.
- Process juice until smooth.
- Before serving, stir it.

Nutritional Benefits:

Bromelain, an enzyme that helps liver detoxification and facilitates digestion, is found in pineapples.
Cilantro is high in chlorophyll and antioxidants, which support liver health and detoxification.
Vitamin C and antioxidants found in lemons shield liver cells from harm.

Greens and Grapefruit Liver Detox Juice

Ingredients:

- 1 peeled grapefruit

- 2 cups of spinach

- 1 cucumber

- 1 cored green apple

- 1-inch slice of ginger

Directions:

- Wash all components thoroughly.
- Peel the grapefruit and ginger.
- Cut the cucumber into smaller pieces if necessary.
- Combine all the ingredients in your juicer.
- Process juice until smooth.
- Before serving, stir it.

Nutritional Benefits:

Antioxidants and vitamin C found in grapefruits help to maintain health and detoxify the liver. Spinach contains antioxidants and chlorophyll, which support liver function and detoxification.

Ginger's anti-inflammatory qualities aid liver function.

Dandelion Detox Green Juice

Ingredients:

- 2 cups of green dandelion

- 1 cucumber

- 2 celery stalks

- 1 cored green apple

- 1/2 lemon, peeled

Directions:

- Wash all components thoroughly.
- Cut the cucumber and apple into smaller pieces if necessary.
- Combine all the ingredients in your juicer.
- Process juice until smooth.
- Before serving, stir it.

Nutritional Benefits:

Dandelion greens promote liver detoxification and bile production, hence facilitating digestion and toxin disposal.

Cucumbers and celery are hydrating and high in antioxidants, which promote liver function.

Apple contains both sweetness and antioxidants, which protect liver cells from harm.

Blueberry Beet Liver Support Juice

Ingredients:

- 1 peeled small beet

- 1 cup of blueberries

- 1/2 cucumber

- 1/2 lemon, peeled

- 1-inch slice of ginger

Directions:

- Wash all ingredients thoroughly.
- Peel the beetroot and lemon.
- Place all the items in your juicer.

- Process juice until smooth.
- Before serving, stir it.

Nutritional Benefits:

Blueberries are high in antioxidants, which help preserve liver cells and improve detoxification.
Beets include betaine, which aids liver cleansing and bile synthesis.
Lemon contains vitamin C and antioxidants that help liver health.

These juicing recipes are specifically designed to benefit liver health by incorporating ingredients high in antioxidants, vitamins, minerals, and other substances that promote detoxification, reduce inflammation, and protect liver cells from harm. Consume these nutritious juices as part of a well-balanced diet to maintain good liver function and general health.

Tips for Creating Your Liver-Health Juice Blend

Making your liver-healthy juice blends allows you to customize recipes based on your taste preferences and ingredient availability while still receiving the advantages of liver-supporting ingredients. Here are some suggestions for making your liver-healthy juice blends.

1. **Choose Liver-Supportive Ingredients**: Consume leafy greens, cruciferous vegetables, beets, citrus fruits, ginger, and turmeric.

2. **Aim for Balance**: Incorporate a variety of flavors, textures, and colors in your juice blends. Combine sweet fruits like apples or oranges with bitter greens like kale or dandelion greens to create a well-rounded flavor profile.

3. **Experiment with Flavor Combinations**: Create unique flavor combinations by combining different components. For a refreshing variation, try adding herbs like

cilantro or mint or spices like cinnamon or cayenne for extra flavor and health benefits.

4. **Consume Citrus**: Citrus fruits such as lemons, limes, oranges, and grapefruits contain vitamin C and flavonoids that promote liver health and detoxification. Citrus can be added to juice mixes for a tart flavor and an additional nutritious boost.

5. **Remember the Greens**: Leafy greens like kale, spinach, and Swiss chard include chlorophyll, antioxidants, and other minerals that aid in liver cleansing and overall wellness. To add nutrients to your juice blends, include a handful of greens.

6. **Use Spices**: Ginger, turmeric, cinnamon, and cayenne pepper not only offer flavor but also have anti-inflammatory and antioxidant characteristics that benefit liver function. Experiment with adding spices to your juice mixes to get more health benefits.

7. **Use Hydrating Ingredients**: Cucumber, celery, and watermelon give volume and freshness to juice mixes while also giving nutrients and supporting liver health.

8. **Consider Nutrient Synergy**: Certain nutrients work together to improve absorption and efficacy. For example, black pepper boosts the absorption of curcumin, the key ingredient in turmeric. Consider using additives that increase vitamin bioavailability in your juice mixes.

9. **Keep it Fresh**: Use fresh, high-quality foods to enhance flavor and nutrition. Choose organic produce to limit your exposure to pesticides and other toxins.

10. **Listen to YourBody**: Pay attention to how your body reacts to various components and combinations. Everyone's taste preferences and nutritional requirements are unique, so tailor your juice blends to your preferences and goals.

By following these guidelines and experimenting with various ingredients and combinations, you may produce delicious and nutritious juice blends that boost liver health and general well-being. Don't be scared to be creative and have fun with your juicing adventures! a healthy juice blend

Chapter 6: Incorporating Juicing into Your Daily Routine

Strategies for Making Juicing a Sustainable Part of Your Lifestyle

Juicing can be an effective tool for improving your health and well-being, but you must discover ways to make it a long-term part of your routine. In this chapter, we'll look at ways to incorporate juicing into your daily routine to ensure long-term success.

I. **Set Realistic Goals**: Set reasonable goals for your juicing adventure. Whether you want to incorporate one juice per day or undertake a juice cleanse once a month, creating attainable goals can help you stay motivated and dedicated.

II. **Establish a Juicing Routine**: Set daily juicing hours to ensure consistency. Whether it's in the morning before breakfast or in the evening after work, having a specific time for juicing will help you develop a habit.

III.   **Plan Ahead**: Prepare your juice recipes and grocery list ahead of time to ensure you have all the necessary items. Preparing ingredients or juices in bulk can also save time and make juicing more convenient.

IV.   **Invest in Quality Equipment**: Choose a juicer that meets your needs and tastes. Select a centrifugal, masticating, or twin-gear juicer that is appropriate for your lifestyle and budget to make juicing a simple and delightful experience.

V.   **Get Creative with Recipes**: Try out different combinations of fruits, veggies, and herbs to make enticing and nourishing juices. To maintain interest and excitement, experiment with different flavors and components.

VI.   **Make it Social**: Invite friends and family to join your juicing journey. Juicing together may be a pleasant and social activity, and having a support network can help you stay accountable and motivated.

VII. **Incorporate Juicing into Meals**: Use fresh juices as a healthy beverage or in smoothies, soups, or salad dressings. This enables you to reap the benefits of juicing while maintaining a healthy diet.

VIII. **Pay Attention to Your Body**: Take note of how your body reacts to juicing and adapt your program accordingly. If juicing in the morning makes you feel better, keep to it. If some ingredients do not agree with you, try different ones.

IX. **Practice Mindfulness**: While juicing, savor each sip and focus on your feelings. Connecting with your body and experiencing juicing can increase your happiness and appreciation for the process.

X. **Maintain Consistency**: Juicing success requires consistency. Even on hectic days or when you're feeling unmotivated, stick to your regimen and make juicing a priority. It will eventually become a natural and effortless part of your existence.

By applying these tactics and making juicing a regular part of your daily routine, you may reap the various health advantages and vivid energy that fresh juices provide. Remember to listen to your body, keep flexible, and enjoy your juicing experience!

How to Balance Juicing with a Healthy Diet

Juicing must be balanced with a healthy diet to ensure that you achieve all of your nutritional requirements while enjoying the benefits of fresh juices. Here are some ideas for reaching this balance:

1. **Promote Whole Foods**: While juicing is a convenient way to consume fruits and vegetables, it's critical to prioritize complete meals in your diet. Whole fruits and vegetables are high in fiber, which is beneficial to digestive health and satiety.

2. **Choose a Variety of Foods:** Include a mix of fruits, vegetables, whole grains, lean meats, and healthy fats in your diet to ensure you obtain a variety of nutrients. Juicing should be used as an addition to your diet rather than as a substitute for full foods.

3. **Consider Portion Proportions**: - While juicing, it's important to pay attention to portion proportions. Fresh juices can be nutrient-dense, but they can also be calorie-dense, especially if they are high in fruit. Consume smaller portions and balance your intake with different foods throughout the day.

4. **Consume Protein and Healthy Fats**: - Including protein and healthy fats in your diet can help regulate blood sugar levels and increase satiety. Nuts, seeds, Greek yogurt, tofu, or avocado can be added to drinks or consumed separately.

5. **Monitor Sugar Content**: Take note of the sugar content in your drinks, especially if they contain a lot of fruit. While natural sugars are

healthier than artificial sugars, eating too much can still influence blood sugar levels. Sweet fruits should be balanced with vegetables, or choose low-sugar options such as berries or green apples.

6. **Customize Your Juice Recipes**: Tailor juice recipes to match your nutritional needs and preferences. Experiment with different combinations of fruits, vegetables, and herbs to produce well-balanced blends that contain a variety of vitamins, minerals, and antioxidants.

7. **Listen to Your Body**: Pay attention to how your body reacts to juicing and adjust your intake accordingly. If you discover that juicing makes you hungry or unsatisfied, try adding more whole foods or protein-rich snacks to your diet.

8. **Stay Hydrated**: Juices can help with hydration, but it's important to drink lots of water throughout the day. Aim to drink at least

eight glasses of water per day to stay hydrated and improve overall health.

9. **Moderation**: Juicing, like any other nutritional component, should be consumed in moderation. Enjoy fresh juices as part of a healthy diet, but don't rely on them only for nourishment.

10. **Consult a Healthcare Expert**: When adopting juicing, consult with a qualified dietitian or healthcare expert about whether you have any special dietary challenges or health conditions.

By following these guidelines and focusing on balance, you can reap the health advantages of juicing while maintaining a well-rounded and healthy diet. Remember that variety, moderation, and listening to your body are all important aspects of a healthy lifestyle.

Monitoring Your Health and Adjusting Your Juicing Practices Accordingly

Monitoring your health is essential when introducing juicing into your lifestyle since it helps you see how your body reacts to changes in your diet. Here are some strategies for tracking your health and altering your juicing habits accordingly:

A. **Regular Check-Ups**: Organize regular check-ups with your healthcare practitioner to monitor your health and discuss dietary and lifestyle adjustments. Your healthcare professional can evaluate your nutritional status, treat any issues, and make personalized recommendations.

B. **Maintain a Food Journal**: - Record your dietary intake, including the types and quantities of juices you consume. Take note of any symptoms or changes in your health, such as changes in energy, digestion, or mood, to uncover trends and potential triggers.

C. **Track Nutrient Intake**: Pay attention to your nutrient consumption, which includes vitamins, minerals, and macronutrients, to ensure that you are reaching your nutritional requirements. Consider working with a trained nutritionist to evaluate your diet and detect any nutrient deficits or imbalances.

D. **Pay Attention to Your Body**: Pay attention to how your body reacts to juicing and alter your habits accordingly. If you experience intestinal pain, fluctuations in energy levels, or other negative effects, you may consider changing your juice recipes, portion amounts, or consumption times.

E. **Adjust Juice Procedures Based on Goals**: Adjust your juicing routine to meet your health goals. If you're juicing for detoxification, weight loss, or a specific health condition, keep track of your progress and make adjustments as needed to maximize your results.

F. **Experiment with Substances**: Try different substances and combinations to see what works best for you. If specific components create bad reactions or allergies, consider removing them from your juices or lowering the amount used.

G. **Stay Hydrated**: Drink adequate water throughout the day, especially if consuming juices. Dehydration can impair your energy levels, digestion, and general health.

H. **Limit Sugar Consumption**: Be cautious of the sugar level in your juices, especially if you have diabetes, insulin resistance, or other metabolic problems. Choose low-sugar fruits and vegetables, and keep your blood sugar levels under control if necessary.

I. **Juice Moderation**: Use juicing sparingly as a supplement to your regular diet. While fresh juices can be healthy, ingesting excessive amounts can result in imbalances and vitamin shortages.

J. **Seek Professional Guidance**: If you have special health issues or dietary restrictions, consult with a certified nutritionist or healthcare provider for personalized suggestions.

By monitoring your health and modifying your juicing methods accordingly, you can ensure that you're getting the most out of your juice routine while also improving your general health and well-being. Remember that everyone's body is unique; therefore, it's important to listen to your body and make modifications that work best for you.

Conclusion

As we near the end of our voyage through the world of juicing for liver health, it becomes clear that we can transform our health. "Juicing for Liver Health: A Guide to Natural Detox and Wellness" offers you the knowledge, tools, and motivation you need to start your journey to better health and energy.

By embracing the healing power of nutrient-rich juices, you've learned how to help your liver's important functions, promote detoxification, and improve your overall health. From nutrient-dense recipes to practical tips for incorporating juicing into your daily routine, you now have the tools you need to take control of your health and recapture your vitality.

But our adventure does not stop here. As you continue your juicing adventure, remember to listen to your body, keep focused on your health goals, and modify your routines as needed. Whether you want to start a better lifestyle, treat specific health conditions, or simply enjoy the benefits of vibrant living, juicing is a powerful and tasty method to nourish your body, mind, and soul.

As you raise your glass to a healthier, happier self, remember that the transformative power of juicing is within grasp. Embrace the journey, savor the flavors, and appreciate the gift of bright health that juicing provides.

Made in the USA
Las Vegas, NV
17 December 2024

14454211R00049